Copyright © 2021 ALISON JAYNE HOUGH

ISBN: 9798507232529

DEDICATION

I DEDICATE THIS BOOK TO MY BROTHER- IN- LAW ANTHONY PHILLIPS WHO DIED SUDDENLY, AGE FIFTY- NINE ON A FISHING TRIP IN FRANCE.

Anthony you were our 'everything'.

Thank you for ringing me the night before you died to tell me how proud you were of me. I wish I had kept you on the telephone for longer. I would give anything just to hear your voice again.

Keep catching those big fish in heaven!

ACKNOWLEDGMENTS

To my dearest husband Steve, you are a blessing, you pick me up when I stumble and always hold me close to your heart.

To my three beautiful children Charlotte, Emily and Christopher who will always be my life's greatest achievements.

To my darling sister Carol who sat beside me, held my hand and helped guide me through this difficult time.

To Mr D Gahir for saving my life!

To Julie for always being there for me and making me whole again

To my amazing home and work friends who sent love, prayers nd best wishes, gifts, food and alcohol!

FOREWARD

I qualified as a nurse in 1986 when I was twenty- one and I have worked in many different areas and specialities of nursing. I have met some very interesting people both patients and staff and my enthusiasm for nursing as a profession has never waned. I now work at a well-respected and highly rated, university as a nurse lecturer and I consider the students I teach, in the same way as the patients/clients I cared for. I encourage them, empower them and invest in them in comparable ways. I feel fortunate to be in this role and I enjoy and value my job immensely.

When I was informed that I had adenocarcinoma of the sinuses on the right side of my face, my nursing experience and knowledge offered some benefit, but mostly I would consider it to be dispiriting as I immediately prophesised the worst outcome. My role now, as a university lecturer involves researching the physical, anatomical, emotional and longevity factors relating to disease, but I avoided investigating my own diagnosis. I can appreciate that many people may feel differently and would prefer to be 'prepared' through knowledge, but I was frightened. I was terrified that I would see an article relating to my type of cancer and find data about poor survival rates following an operation, or high, short term mortality rates. I felt that this evidence may have affected my response to cancer and attitude regarding the surgery and treatment. I considered that I needed to preserve the degree of optimism and confidence I held in the hope that I may recover.

This book cites my experience of having cancer from diagnosis to treatment and beyond. It also includes discussion about how the people already present in my life or who entered my life as a result of my diagnosis, supported me in different ways. There are some brief paradigms from my childhood which I include to illustrate perhaps, how I was able to have the resilience and resolve to manage this difficult journey. I have written from the perspective of 'me' as a patient and not 'me' as a nurse thus avoiding the use of technical jargon which I think may detract from the depth and intensity of my reactions and emotions. I do not consider that everyone's experience of cancer will be the same as mine, this is personal to me but there may be some elements within my 'story' which are identifiable to others.

This memoir is an unembellished, real life, raw, gritty, sometimes sad and sometimes humorous portrayal of my actual experiences.

INTRODUCTION

Prior to writing this memoir I thought long and hard about the concept of cancer, its connotations, effects and association with me. Cancer seems a strange word, almost onomatopoetic in that it sounds like what it is; destructive, menacing, diseased and corruptive. I struggle, even today to correlate myself with this terminology and avoid it by using descriptors such as 'my illness' or 'when I was unwell.'

I have also read about people describing their experience of having cancer as a '*battle*' or '*fight*' and I can relate to this but what did it mean to me? Writing retrospectively of course, these terms seemed a little too aggressive. I did not consider cancer to be something which I needed to *battle* or *fight*. My approach was to acknowledge it, understand it, even revere it a little and then move forwards with or without it. Of course, I held a degree of contempt towards the effect it had on me, my family and my friends but I did not feel any anger or abhorrence.

People with cancer are also often portrayed by others as '*suffering or enduring*' cancer, expressions which completely contrast with '*battling or fighting.*' These terms sound a little too '*wretched*' and '*self-defeating*'. '*Challenge, test, confront and face*' seem to sit in the middle for me. These words could signify something good or not so good. They acknowledge that the person with cancer could still be in the 'driving seat', and that whilst life can be straight forward it also presents obstacles which must be *managed*. The *challenge* presented by cancer is not easy, but it is also not always permeated by doom and gloom. Cancer can also present some unique experiences which may change one's way of thinking, of behaving and of living life.

1: THE SYMPTOMS

In March 2016 Steve and I took an early spring holiday to Tenerife. We had a fabulous time soaking up the sun, drinking prosecco and fine dining. We had been married for almost thirty years and we felt secure and happy with life. We had three adult 'children' for whom we had spent many years nurturing, engaging them in activities such as sports, music, swimming, drama and horse riding and taken an active interest in their education. When they were very young, we bought a small holding in the country to enable them to have pets such as geese, goats, chickens, horses and sheep and to enable them to enjoy a happy, outdoor life with their friends. They had now all 'flown the nest,' secured well paid employment and loving partners endorsing their financial and emotional independence. As usually quite modest people we did feel therefore that we should give each other a 'pat on the back.'

Well! the saying is that *'pride comes before a fall*!' and this was certainly my experience!

We returned from our holiday in Tenerife, and I had a congested nose and a sore throat. I considered that it may have been due to the inflight air conditioning but following weeks of congestion I decided to visit my General Practitioner (GP). I was then, without any medical assessment! diagnosed with sinusitis and prescribed antibiotics and a nasal spray. I felt confident with the diagnosis but two weeks later, following no relief from the medication, I arranged another appointment. I was again, not examined but I was prescribed a different course of antibiotics and nasal drops and asked to return if the symptoms persisted.

As the weeks passed, I began to find it difficult to eat as one side of my nose was now constantly blocked. I had to eat with my mouth open and chewing even small amounts of food was literally exhausting! If I tried to breathe through the unblocked nostril, it acted almost like a vacuum and flattened to the middle of my nose thus preventing any air from entering. I also developed a relentless, dull headache which made me feel tired and irritable. One Friday evening, I went upstairs to lie down for a short period, and I started to cry. I was feeling rather sorry for myself as I was exhausted from lack of sleep due to the congestion and I struggled to focus on anything due to the nauseating, continual headache. As I cried, I suddenly became aware of a lot of fluid coming out of my mouth. At first, I thought that it was an increase in saliva due to the tears and my blocked nose but as I looked down, I saw a huge amount of blood. The blood was draining of my mouth rather than my nose (as it would with a nose- bleed) and some of the blood was clotting at the back of my throat. I was afraid that the clots would occlude my only airway and I began to panic. I banged on the bedroom floor to gain my husband's attention and after seeing me choking and struggling to breathe he rang the emergency services. They attended promptly and advised that I should go with them to the hospital. I was reluctant, because the bleeding had ceased, and I felt much calmer and so after observing me for some time the paramedics left but urged me to make an appointment with my GP as soon as possible.

I lay in bed 'propped up' with pillows that night, terrified that the bleeding may start again. I was afraid to sneeze or cough in case the pressure initiated a further bleed and I began to worry that my symptoms could be indicative of something more serious than sinusitis. On the Monday I requested an urgent appointment with the GP to inform them of the posterior nosebleed, and continued congestion. Despite my attempts at assertiveness, I felt that the GP did not take my concerns seriously, and I was again prescribed different antibiotics and an alternative nasal spray. I left feeling frustrated and very unwell, but I went back to work as I needed to attend a meeting. I apologised for my lateness and gave a brief precis of the reason. I sat down, and then almost immediately I stood up. I made my excuses and walked out of the room, and down the corridor toward my office. It was at this point that I realised how ill I was feeling. I had a nauseating headache and I felt weak and faint. I stumbled past my manager's office to the safe- haven of my office so that I could sit in darkness. My manager however, had followed me and after some discussion she instructed me to go home. She advised me to make another appointment with a different doctor as soon as possible, advice that normally I would have been able to ascertain for myself, but my brain felt so fuzzy and confused. I drove home (which I probably should not have) in a complete haze; I barely remember the journey and it was almost as if the car had steered me home by itself.

Like my father, I had a strong work ethic and I hated to take time off for illness, but I knew that I could not return to work until I had some answers as to why I felt so ill. I had never felt so sure about a decision and it was strangely empowering. When I arrived home, I took off my coat, placed my handbag on a chair and went upstairs to rest on my bed and it was in my bed that I stayed for a whole week. I took analgesia for my headache and telephoned the doctors surgery to implore them to refer me to see a hospital specialist. Later that week however I knew that I could not wait for an appointment. I could see a 'growth' protruding from my right nostril. It was white and grey and it felt hard and dry. I panicked a little and asked Steve to look at it. He thought that it looked a little like an ulcer and his appeasing approach made me feel a little more composed. Despite this I sought advice from a friend's husband who was an Ear, Nose and Throat (ENT) consultant. It was not a decision I had taken lightly because I did not want to place him in a difficult situation however when I sent a photograph of the 'growth' to him he was concerned and an appointment was made for me to see a hospital specialist and undergo a Computerised Tomography (CT) scan.

2: THE APPOINTMENT

On the day of the Ear Nose and Throat (ENT) appointment, my husband and I were asked to take a seat in a waiting room full of parents and children. I thought that this was a little odd as I expected to see other adults looking and feeling as ill as me. After a short period of time my name was announced, and my husband and I entered the clinical room, where there was a doctor and a health care support worker (HCSW). The doctor asked a few questions about my symptoms and nodded repetitively and rather too quickly as I answered. He mentioned the word sinusitis and his verbal and non -verbal communication made me feel that he was not too concerned. I began to feel a little confused, surely, he must have read the referral letter from my friend's husband. I then mentioned that I had had a CT scan and he looked surprised. I concluded then that this appointment was as a result of the GP referral and that this was a routine ENT clinic appointment rather than an urgent one. He turned his chair away from me to access his computer and the results of the scan and it was at this point that everything changed. He fell silent, looked shocked and then took a deep breath. I could see that this was not something that he was expecting to have to manage during his regular clinic schedule. His very profound facial expression made me feel tense and anxious, I felt my whole body tighten and I sat motionless, hardly daring to breathe. He turned his chair towards me, leant forward and looked at me with concern etched across his face. He spoke softly and with unease as he gave details about the results of the scan. He then turned the computer screen so that my husband and I could see it and there was a picture of the frontal part of my skull, head and neck. The left side of my face showed numerous black areas which illustrated the air within my sinuses. The right side of my face revealed a mirror skeletal image but instead of black air spaces they were totally white. There was no air within the sinuses on the right side of my face. The doctor told my husband and I that the scan was of significant concern and that the white areas indicated 'some type of growth'.

It was then that I asked him in a very shaky and panicky voice if I had cancer. I did not look at his expression as I felt that this would confirm my worst fears.

He told me that '*the growth*' could be any number of things and that I would need a biopsy to confirm a diagnosis. There was no conviction in his voice that all was well, he looked resigned somehow as if he already knew that it *was* serious. He offered me no reassuring words and he seemed slightly anguished and sorrowful. He spoke about "*lots of swollen blood vessels at the back of my nose which were liable to bleed again*" and so *he* advised me to try to refrain from blowing my nose, sneezing, crying or coughing. My husband repeated these words to me after we had left the hospital, as I had not even heard them. My mind was in a stupor, a fog. I felt as if all my blood had drained away from my body and I leant forward placing my head in my hands as if to support myself. I felt numb and detached from the situation. I remember saying "*I can't die!*" "*I'm only fifty -two and my daughter is getting married in April next year*". I could not believe that I was saying these words, they seemed so out of context, unbelievable and disconnected from me and my life. This cannot be happening I thought! My voice also sounded different, it lacked strength and assertion. I heard a noise and looked around to see the HCSW wiping tears from her eyes! "*This is the worst part of my job*" she sniffed. I could not understand why she was upset. This could not be because of me! My head felt as if it was full of cotton wool and I had no thought processes which would enable me to make sense of this situation. The HCSW then ushered Steve and I into a small room opposite the clinical room. She sat down, but we did not. Steve and I stood like statues, frozen in time and motion, unable to speak, think, cry, scream, walk or run. The HCSW asked if we would like a cup of tea and I shook my head and quietly thanked her for the offer. My eyes diverted toward a small, faded artificial flower arrangement situated on a round coffee table in the centre of the room. This is the room where they bring people to impart difficult or bad news or to offer comfort I thought. Cheap, low uncomfortable chairs, a basic, round coffee table in the middle of the room, a faded artificial flower arrangement and a box of tissues. I fleetingly recalled the irony of the situation in that as a qualified nurse I too had led grieving or anxious relatives into similar rooms to help support them following difficult situations. Now this was me! I was in '*the room*' the impact of the environment had somehow failed me a nurse. Then it had seemed to have been an unassuming, quiet space, a place of comfort. Now it felt as if I was in God's waiting room, I was a detainee in a new realm which I did not wish to be part of.

After declining the tea and not opting to sit down or ask any questions, Steve and I were escorted to the pre-operative assessment unit. Here, my height, weight, blood pressure, pulse and an ECG were recorded to assess whether I was well enough to have a general anaesthetic. The routine investigations were confirmed to be within a normal range. I was healthy enough to pass the health assessment and yet I could be dying I mused. This awful concept kept whirling around in my head. I already felt defeated, I had no positive thoughts, just absolute despair. Steve and I exited the hospital and we drove to a small park where we sat on a bench. We had not yet spoken to eachother, we were too embroiled in our own thoughts. I looked around and saw parents with children and babies in pushchairs, dogs running after sticks and elderly people walking hand in hand. I remember thinking how can life be so 'normal' for other people when it is destroying me?

3: DEATH AND DYING

I was brought up in a modest semi-detached house on the outskirts of a small market town with my mother, father and elder sister Carol. Carol and I had a friend, Sandra and the three of us would often visit the corner shop owned by Mrs Simpson who looked to be about a hundred years old (she was probably only about sixty!). She was a small, shrivelled, grumpy woman who wore glasses which were precariously perched onto her rather large nose. Sandra would ask for the half penny chew box which was situated under the counter and Mrs Simpson would tut and groan as she bent down to retrieve the box. As soon as she had stooped down out of sight, we would all grab a handful of the two pence chews (which were in cardboard boxes on the top of the counter) and stuff them quickly into our pockets. Mrs Simpson was suspicious of our antics but accepted our halfpennies with a grumble and we would then leave. I can still remember the sound of the bell as the shop door closed. We continued with this immoral activity until one day my mother entered our bedroom with a very stern look on her face. She informed us that 'someone' had seen us go into Mrs Simpsons shop with no money and come out with lots of sweets. We never questioned the logic of this statement and assumed later, (as we got older) that she was trying to be tactful and gentle with her accusation. We immediately blamed our behaviour on Sandra, who was not present to defend herself, thinking that this may help the situation as my mother disliked Sandra and called her *'that naughty girl'* Despite our plea mother instructed us to empty our piggy banks and take the money to the shop to pay for the sweets we had stolen. I remember feeling very ashamed of my behaviour and vowed never to steal sweets again. One year later, when I was about nine years old two local boys informed me that, Mrs Simpson had died *(whilst sitting on the toilet).*

"The fire brigade had to bust her door down and drag her skeleton out of the bathroom!"

One local boy exclaimed, rather too excitedly.

I remember being horrified about this. Poor Mrs Simpson had died whilst 'sitting on the toilet' how awful! And how embarrassing! I also recall feeling unnerved at the thought of her being alone dying and her consequent death. This was the first time that I really thought about my own mortality and it felt quite overwhelming. I reconciled myself with the thought that only old people die, and I had my whole life ahead of me. This concept, however, was tested when I was at junior school and in a whole school assembly it was announced that a girl in the year above me had died. It was my sister's friend and she had died suddenly of an asthma attack. I remember that some children laughed, out loud, right there in the assembly hall! I understand now that they were too young to fully comprehend the concept of death and its finality and that their laughter was just another ill placed emotion, which would have been reflexive rather than uncaring. I, in contrast, remember sitting there quietly surrounded by a room full of people yet feeling alone and bewildered.

When Steve and I returned home following the consultation those feelings of loneliness and bewilderment returned. Despite knowing how much Steve loved me and that he too was worried about my diagnosis and resulting prognosis I knew that I was the one who potentially had cancer and that I was the one who may die. I was, and still am afraid of dying. I do not want to die, I am fearful of dying, and I do not want to leave the people I love behind. I had and still have enough knowledge and life experience to make this judgement and I am not sure that my perspective will ever change.

As time progressed, I became even more convinced that I would die. How would I die? What would happen when I died? Would I know that I was dying? What would I see and hear? What would I feel? As a nurse, I had sat beside and comforted many people who were dying. Many of them were heavily sedated and would just, take their last breath and then 'fade away' with no drama. They had 'gone' no one would hear their voices again, their laughter, appreciate their personalities and their life experiences. Their bodies lay still, pale and cool to touch. Would this be me?

I also felt sad that life would continue without me. Retrospectively it seems quite a selfish point of view but Steve was only in his fifties. He could meet someone else, love someone else and share this other person with our children. Birthdays and Christmas's would continue without me and I would never get to see my future grand-children, or my daughter and son get married. These thoughts and feelings were all encompassing, and very difficult to manage. It took time before I resigned myself to the fact that there was absolutely nothing that I could do to change the situation I was in. This was not an acceptance. I knew that I would never fully accept that I could die. I just had to try to cope with the possibility.

4: TELLING OUR 'GROWN UP CHILDREN'

The worst part, for me, was informing Charlotte, Emily and Christopher about the details of the appointment and the need for a biopsy. They all knew that we were attending the hospital and I suspected that the tone of Steve's voice when he rang them, would prompt them to think that bad news was coming. Steve suggested that we invite them to our house so that we could inform them together. I knew that I would have to ring Emily as she lived in North Wales and I would not want her to drive to our house in a worried state.

Whilst recounting this experience, I have tears in my eyes. I felt then, as I still do, so terribly guilty and sad. I knew that they would all find this information so incredibly difficult, and I did not want to affect their lives in a way that I knew would hurt them. The uncertainty we would all have to endure until we got the results of the biopsy would be hard for us to manage. The language used and the way that I am writing this seems so formal and yet every word is filled with emotion. I know that we are not unique in stating that we feel that our children are beautiful people both inside and out. That they are clever, self-sufficient, loving and caring. They mean everything to Steve and I and yet, whilst they remain blissfully unaware, we must hurt them by giving them information, which is likely to affect their feelings of security and happiness. It was heart-breaking. I have no other way of describing it.

Charlotte appeared first and ran up the driveway to the small conservatory where Steve and I were sitting. She looked distressed and anxious for information, but we had to wait for Christopher who appeared shortly afterward. I was as honest and detailed as I could be when I informed them about the consultation and the way forward in terms of the biopsy. I did not want to leave any scope for confusion or error in the information presented. They sat quietly and listened as Steve and I had done during the consultation. They looked crestfallen, pale and worried. They asked no questions and looked at the floor as if they were trying to comprehend what was being said. I was relieved that neither of them stated that the biopsy may reveal something less sinister because I did not feel that I could reassure them or defend my fears without crying.

Charlotte displayed a mixture of emotions. Initially there were tears, then frustration and slight anger toward the circumstance she had found herself in. I put my arms around her to help comfort her and I wished that I could change things and make them better as I had done when she was a little girl. My arms held her tightly as I did not wish to 'let her go'. I wanted to absorb her pain, but I knew that I could not. I knew that there was nothing that I could do to protect them both from this situation we had all found ourselves in. Words of reassurance would have been futile, erroneous and somehow cruel. Christopher was more stoic. He internalised a lot of his feelings, but his face was etched in sadness. I was aware that he had suspected '*the worst*' a few weeks previously as he had been researching my symptoms on the internet. He was the youngest of the three and I desperately wanted to protect him. I reached out and held him close. His body was tense, and I suspected that he was trying to be brave. I felt a surge of absolute devastation. I desperately wanted to cry but I was so afraid that this may cause another posterior nose- bleed and upset Charlotte and Christopher even more.

Ringing Emily was also very difficult. She was out walking her dog, Walter, with a close friend and initially she sounded happy to hear my voice. I so desperately wanted to cry but I knew that I had to be strong for her so that I could comfort her and help her to believe that I was managing the situation. I spoke to her gently and summarised the details without leaving any key information out. I heard her crying quietly and I felt as if my heart would break. My body was full of pain and anguish and it hurt so badly. I had to walk up and down the garden at quite a fast pace to prevent myself from falling to the ground and crying. I so desperately wanted to wrap my arms around her, hold her tight and kiss her. I felt that she was my little girl again, not the beautiful, confident young woman she had become. It was so incredibly traumatic. She whispered goodbye and left me feeling that I needed to go to Wales and see her, but I knew that her partner Dean would support her and that there was absolutely nothing I could do to make the situation any easier.

Emily was planning her wedding and it should have been such a happy time for her. I felt so guilty that I had impacted so negatively on this precious time, I blamed myself and in the emotion which also embodied me in such a prolific way was sadness in a way that I had never experienced before.

I am quite pragmatic by nature and not usually driven by emotion. Finding and expressing the words which would inform my children of the possibility of me having cancer was by far one of the worst things I have had to do. The pain I felt reflected only that of when my father died. The finality, the destruction of a once happy existence and the realisation that nothing will ever be the same, seemed huge, insurmountable hurdles.

The results of the biopsy were disseminated to my family and I at home via telephone which I placed on 'loud speak' on the table so that everyone could hear what was being said and ask questions accordingly.

I advised everyone that they should leave the room if the information was too difficult for them to hear. My eldest daughter Charlotte sat stoically taking notes as the consultant spoke. Emily intermittently shed tears quietly, and Christopher stood by the door of the room looking solemn and Steve looked pale and anxious.

The consultant confirmed our worst fears: the biopsy had revealed a stage 4 adenocarcinoma of the sinuses and it occupied every available space in the right side of my nose, sinuses and behind my right eye and upward, very close to the margin of my brain. We were informed that if I had waited two weeks longer it would have penetrated the meninges (protective covering of the brain) and I would have a terminal prognosis. Whilst the diagnosis had not been a revelation to me, I had never lost hope of receiving a more favourable result and so it was an incredible shock.

5: I SHOULD HAVE MY OWN CHAIR!

Prior to the operation I had a further CT, Magnetic Resonance Imaging (MRI) and a Positron Emission Tomography (PET) scan. It was a huge relief to be told that the cancer had not spread but I was informed that there was only a small, cancer free margin near to my brain. Time was clearly of the essence and so I had to attend the hospital two or three times every week for various consultations. At every appointment I was given even more difficult information. I was informed that the surgery would require the expertise of four consultants: a maxillary facial consultant, a neurologist (as the tumour was very close to my brain) an ear, nose and throat consultant and an orthodontic consultant. The maxillary facial consultant (Mr Gahir) was a tall, handsome man with perfect white teeth and a soft voice. He examined my right eye carefully and then explained that I had exophthalmos which meant that my eye was 'bulging' outwards due to the pressure of the tumour. This was not something I had noticed, but it seemed to add weight to the diagnosis that I had been given and the headaches that I had been experiencing. I was told incrementally that I would lose my right eye, whole nose and part of my right cheek. Mr Gahir explained that a less radical approach would not save my life and even this major 'line of attack' may not guarantee my long- term survival. I consented to the extreme method of surgery acknowledging that anything less compromising may result in my demise.

If I wanted to live, I had to take the opportunity that I was being offered. This destructive, life threatening tumour had not only invaded the significant features of the right side of my face, but it had also compromised my very being and eradicated the confidence I had taken for granted regarding my health status. I firmly believed that my body had 'let me down,' I did not drink excessively or smoke, I was relatively active and ate a healthy diet. This cancer had exposed a vulnerability in me which I had not encountered before and initially isolated me from the person that I thought I was.

Alongside the tough reality of the fundamentals of the operation however, Mr Gahir spoke with optimism. He informed me that he would be placing implants into the bone around my face and forehead and that later the magnets at the end of the implants would be 'charged' to enable a magnetic prosthetic nose, eye and part cheek to be situated, firmly over the cavity. These innovative strategies would he hoped, enable me to feel and look more confident in the future. As the weeks prior to the operation progressed the trust I felt for him grew. He was so intelligent, so patient centred and so personable. I had every confidence that he would try his best to save my life and ensure that my future would be manageable.

I also found great comfort in the support offered to me by Julie who was a Maxillary facial technician. We had met on the day that the extent of the operation was explained to my family and I. Julie explained that after the operation she would be able to make me a prosthetic nose and cheek and eventually an eye. I felt an instant connection with Julie. She was easy to talk to and her expertise and explanation of how the prosthetics would be made gave me an enormous sense of hope.

My focus at prior to this point however was on the operation, I had not really considered what would happen post-operatively. I knew that I would lose my eye, nose and part of my cheek but I had not even thought about what this would look like and what it may mean for my future emotional well- being.

6: THE DAY BEFORE!

On the day before the operation, I went to the cemetery to visit my father's grave. I took flowers and spoke aloud asking him to 'look after me during the surgery' My father had been a great role model and blessing in my life, and it gave me a sense of comfort to be able to be alone there at the cemetery '*with him.*' I kissed his gravestone before I left and I felt a sense of reassurance. I believed that he was with me and that I would be safe in his care.

My Father

My father had been a tall, good looking, strong man who, for most of his working career had been employed as a nurse. He had an artificial leg due to a motor bike accident he had when he was very young. Despite this and the discomfort he often felt, he had an exemplary sickness record, and he encouraged my sister and I to follow his work ethic which meant not succumbing to minor illness. This included of course that absence from school was not an option unless we were requiring a visit to the General Practitioner (GP) or Emergency/Accident Unit. My father adopted an authoritarian parenting style (which was popular in the sixties and seventies) and he would often state '*you do as I say and not as I do*' which my sister and I did not dare to disagree with. The boundaries he set however, were intelligent, clear and coherent leaving no element for confusion or error. This style of parenting (whilst leaving little opportunity for developing self- confidence, problem solving or creating personal choices) helped to embed worthy morals and values within my persona. My father made me feel safe and loved.

My father died many years before my diagnosis of cancer, and this created a huge emotional and physical omission for me. He would have offered a sense of perspective and stability to my fragile state, particularly when I first had my diagnosis. Instead, I had to think about what he would say and how he would guide me.

My strength and resolve also came, in part from my best friend Sharon. I met her when I was thirteen as she had moved into a house opposite my house. Several days after her family had settled into their home, I plucked up the courage to visit her. She was in the garden with her father and I asked her if she wanted to 'hang out' with me. Sharon informed me in a quite surly tone that she was 'too busy propagating cacti and succulents. I had no idea what she was talking about! and so I turned on my heels and left rather hastily. Several seconds later she was by my side and there she has stayed for the past forty-four years. We held the same beliefs and values and together we learned to problem solve, assert ourselves and take minor risks which enabled us to 'grow up' cognitively as well as physically. Sharon's vivid red hair and fiery temperament both terrified and captivated me however during one minor conflict Sharon informed me that she did not like my boyfriend as he had 'sly eyes!' He did actually! But I retorted rather spitefully that her boyfriend had a 'fish face.' This retaliation was empowering and gave me the aptitude in a more mature way of course to object and interject with other's when I felt that I needed to.

I still question my lack of assertiveness when I visited the General Practitioner prior to my diagnosis. I can only determine that this may have been because although I may have suspected that my illness was something more serious than sinusitis maybe I was not ready to accept that it could be cancer. It seems so profound to me that I did not ask the General practitioner to assess me properly or that I would accept yet another course of antibiotics and nasal spray. My voice and my opinion were not listened to which is concerning but perhaps I was not assertive enough and I still have no idea why. Whilst the outcome would not have changed it may have offered me an earlier hospital appointment leaving less time for me to worry and become so unwell.

Religion.

From a very young age Carol and I went to church every Sunday and when we were young teenagers' we became altar servers. The church was a 'high church' and the service was long and wordy. I tried to make sense of the sermon and the verses within the bible, but I often struggled to relate them to the life that I was living. Despite this I prayed to God and Jesus the night before my operation. I asked them to take care of me. I promised that if they 'let me live' then I would strive to be a better person.

On the day before the operation my family and I also visited the vicar who had married Charlotte the previous year. He said a prayer for us all and I became a little tearful. I felt utterly overcome with emotion, but I was determined to stay strong. I knew that if lost control of my feelings I would have struggled to regain control of them. The vicar advised me that just before the anaesthetic 'takes hold' I should,

"try to picture where you will be and how you will feel, in that moment when all is well."

He suggested that I should also think about the *"sounds, smells and vista of the imagined place"*.

As soon as I got home, I walked into the field at the back of my house and looked all around me. The field was slightly elevated from the adjoining land enabling me to see a good distance ahead. There was beauty all around me. Features that I had seen on many occasions but now I was looking at them with more clarity. The fields ahead had so many different tones of green as did the hedges. The sky looked almost biblical with its dense fluffy, white clouds. I could feel the breeze on my face and smell the grass and wild flowers in the air. This is what I would think about tomorrow. I did not need anything grand like a beach in Barbados or a port in Monaco. This was a part of my everything, this was 'normal life' my life, my home, my field, my life and I loved it!

7: THE DAY OF THE OPERATION & CRITICAL CARE

On the day of the operation Steve escorted me to the surgical admissions ward. The three other consultants joined Mr Gahir, Steve and I to clarify the main elements of the operation and the expected time it would take, (which was approximately seventeen hours). I readily signed the consent form and inwardly acknowledged that if I wanted to live this was my only option which gave me a sense of acceptance. The consultants left and when Steve wrapped his arms around me to kiss me and say goodbye, I became a little teary.

It felt like such a precious moment. I had known Steve since I was seventeen, he was my strength, he was my everything, our two souls were so connected and sharing this experience had bonded us even more deeply. When he left, I silently said a prayer for us both. I prayed that all the cancer would be removed, and that we would not be separated at this time, through death.

I changed into a theatre gown and pulled the long, green elastic stockings onto my legs. These stockings would hopefully prevent me from getting a blood clot due to the long period of immobility I would sustain during and after the operation. I felt like a patient then, I looked like every other person on the ward. Part of my identity lay in the clothes that I had worn when I had arrived at the hospital and they were now folded away neatly into a bag. I also felt a little vulnerable and submissive. I had done everything the nurses and consultants had requested of me to prepare for this operation and now I knew that I had very little control over the scheduled processes. I did however have full confidence in the surgeons who would be operating and I was grateful for the opportunity that they had afforded me. I knew that they could instead have considered the grade, size and type of tumour to be inoperable and as such decided to treat me palliatively. The anaesthetist came to visit and made me laugh as he asked me what alcoholic drink I would like prior to the anaesthetic. I replied that I would like a Gin and Tonic to which he further enquired as to the type of Gin I liked and whether a lemon or lime would be my favourite garnish. Although I never drink Gin and Tonic, I responded with the first thing that popped into my head. We then had a further discussion about it as he gave me the anaesthetic, and that was the last thing I recall.

Following the operation, I spent several days in critical care. My family visited and Carol spent many hours sitting by my bedside and helping to care for me. I remember little of this time except that very early in the post-operative period my senses, particularly hearing and touch were heightened. This meant that when Carol stroked my arm as a means of reassurance it felt like a thousand needles were being prodded into me. Voices which were calling my name or giving me information sounded too loud and jolted me from my almost inert state. Of course, I was so heavily sedated that I could not move or speak. When I was a little more responsive, I remember a doctor asking me a few neurological assessment questions such as, *'do you know where you are?'* *'who is the Queen of England?'* and finally *'what year is it?'* I was able to answer the first two questions, but I paused as I tried to remember the current year. I remember saying 1986 to which the doctor replied *'that'll do'* I heard him laugh quietly as he walked away and realised that I had made an error. I also recall that the nurses providing my personal care were very kind, and encouraging stating words such as; *'well done Alison,'* or *'you are doing so well.'* I also heard *'this must be very difficult for you'* which made me feel that I was being treated with dignity and respect.

I remember a particularly difficult time when the feeding tube which was going through my nose and into my stomach had somehow dislodged. I vomited profusely and I was also choking. The nurse in charge of my care was using suction and requesting that the ventilation should be removed. It was a tense time, and I was quite traumatised by it. Despite this, Carol, who was still by my side was fabulous. She kept reassuring me that '*everything will be alright*' in a calm and controlled manner. The trust I had in her to help to look after me was unrivalled and enabled me to remain composed and prevent me from panicking. Carol was the only person in my life who had known me for every day of my life. She was able therefore to reassure me in a way that no one else could. Carol did everything she could to care for me and protect me.

The nurses and Carol also kept a journal which would (when I recovered) help to fill the void for the days I had 'missed' whilst I was sedated. Carol also pasted emails into the journal from my friends and work colleagues. It took several months before I felt strong enough to read the journal but when I did, I found messages from Charlotte, Emily, Christopher and Steve about the days and times that they visited me and notes about my treatment and care from my key nurse. Reading these messages helped me to 'make sense' of the experience I had in hospital which in turn enabled me to '*move forwards*' on my journey.

8: ALISON IN WONDERLAND!

After three days in critical care, I was transferred to a ward and nursed in a side room. I had still not looked at myself in a mirror, but I could sense that there were a lot of dressings on my face, and a rudimentary, rather large prosthetic nose.

I was still on quite a lot of strong medication and the effects of this were also quite bizarre. I could visualise a large 'map' on the wall in front of me. It was a map of the streets of Birmingham. I could move the map from side to side with my remaining eye and I saw lots of buildings, roads and houses but I could not make out the street names. I am unfamiliar with the city of Birmingham; I only know New Street Railway Station and so I was a little perplexed as to why I could see all the streets in this particular city. I then saw a large photograph of a black Labrador. It was on the same wall as the 'map' had been. It was static but kept appearing and disappearing alongside an old black and white photograph of a little girl. The images did not unsettle me as they held no relevance to me or my past.

I also believed that I could still see out of my absent right eye. If a nurse entered my room on the right side of me, I could still 'see' them long after they had gone. In addition, their movements were repetitive for example, if the nurse changed an intravenous fluid bag, I could see their arm moving up and down rhythmically and continually for many minutes.

The 'moving images' ceased and were replaced by more static but vivid visualisations. I 'saw' a child hiding behind my door, she was a pretty, little Asian girl about five years old. I heard her 'mother calling her' and I kept shouting *'she's here, she's here'*. The child was looking at me and holding her finger to her lips as if to tell me to be quiet. I thought I should inform the nurse, so I pressed my call bell and explained the situation. I heard her say '*I think I need to speak to the doctor about the amount of medication you are on*' I remember thinking *'what a strange response.'*

After approximately one week the visual and auditory hallucinations ceased but my brain remained 'muddled.' I could not work out the layout of the room. The door (which was to the bathroom) seemed as if it opened into the main ward and I was a little concerned that other patients may come into my room. In addition, I could see out onto the main corridor of the ward it looked wide, uncluttered and devoid of people but when the physiotherapists assisted me to walk down this same corridor, I did not recognise it. It was busy with nurses, doctor's and therapists. Equipment lined the corridor and a large nurses' station occupied its centre.

"My overall goal" I stated one day to the physiotherapists *"is to walk over to the patio doors in my room and sit out on the balcony"* I saw them look at each other with a puzzled expression and then one of them said; *"you are four floors up on a neurology ward, I don't think it would be safe to have a balcony". That is just an ordinary window."* I laughed as I could understand how ridiculous this must have sounded and they laughed with me.

As I became slightly more lucid, I recollect feeling almost euphoric. I was so happy to be still alive following such a large operation and I was also relieved that the weeks of pre-operative preparation were over. I did not know at this point how much of the tumour the surgeons had managed to extract but I was just grateful that I was 'on the other side of things.' This elation has never really left me but at its peak, during my hospital recovery I felt as If I could climb

Mount Everest! I was chatty and positive and would engage enthusiastically in any of the recommended physical exercises, fluid and nutrition requirements advised. As soon as I was able, I was out of bed showering, washing my hair and sitting in a chair. One day a consultant and a junior doctor, who I was not familiar with came to see me and asked me how I was feeling. Following my rather too exuberant response I heard the consultant, inform the junior doctor about the rarity of the tumour that I had. The consultant then glanced at me as she spoke, I was sitting in my chair with a huge smile on my face! I have no idea what either person thought about my mannerisms, perhaps they considered it to be the effects of the medication, but it was not, I was genuinely happy.

9: OTHER PEOPLE'S PERCEPTIONS OF ME

One day a member of the domestic staff (who I had not met before) gave me tea in a plastic sipper cup. As I spoke, she jumped a little. I presumed that she thought that I could not see or talk. I explained that I would prefer an ordinary teacup, to which she willingly obliged. This event made me smile but also consider how some people automatically make assumptions without exploring the reality of a situation. These assumptions may be something that I would have to manage. Would people think that I had been in a fire or a road traffic incident, would they look at me with pity or disdain? If they asked me what had happened to me, what would I say?

A hairdresser came to visit from the salon attached to the hospital. She offered me a wide range of headbands which would help disguise the shaven area of my head and she informed me that I would be able to choose a wig from the salon if my hair 'fell out' as a result of radiotherapy. This offered me strategies I could use to help myself adjust to the current and potential change in my appearance. To her astonishment however, without using a mirror I pulled the headband straight over the top of my dressings, and almost dislodged my nose. It was then that I decided to see how the headband looked and determine if it needed any adjustment. I leapt off the bed and walked quickly into the bathroom and sat down in front of quite a large mirror. I laughed completely spontaneously and somewhat frenziedly at my reflection in the mirror. The temporary prosthetic nose reminded me of a large pig snout and wisps of my once quite thick hair were sticking out randomly from the top of my shaven head. My chin and remaining cheek were also swollen. I felt embarrassed that I had looked like this whilst I had chatted to ward staff and the visitors I had received. My thought was that I resembled something from a horror movie. I looked hideous! The headband did little to help and so I took it off. The hairdresser reassured me that I may wish to wear it once the bandages had been removed. She then exited the room rather swiftly, leaving me to consider the somewhat 'over the top' response I had expressed during her visit.

On another day, a counsellor visited me. The counsellor, a woman, was equally as attractive as the hairdresser had been and I smiled inwardly at the irony of this. Here I was looking and feeling like some sort of strange caricature and there she was looking as if she had stepped off a page from Vogue magazine. It was soon clear however, that she was both professional and very caring. She spoke to me in a soft and calm manner advising me that if I felt I needed support when I was discharged home then she would be there for me. I responded positively to this suggestion thinking that in the long term this may be of benefit. She said goodbye and I was left contemplating the enormity of the adjustments I had to make to help preserve my emotional wellbeing.

During my hospital stay the ENT consultant who had been part of the team who had operated on me came to visit. He pulled up a chair to sit by my bedside. I thought this was a little unusual as consultant visits are usually quite short and concise. He asked me how I was feeling and if I felt that I would 'cope' when I got home. He told me about a man who had, had a similar operation but when he was discharged from hospital he struggled to accept or manage the changes to his face and he had to be admitted to a psychiatric ward. 'Yes,' I thought to myself, I can understand this man's anguish, but I simply said that I would be fine. He informed me that he was hopeful that all of the tumour had been removed but that he could not be sure until the bone samples had been examined to determine whether there was a healthy enough margin between the removed bone and my brain. To my surprise he then became a little tearful as he recounted that as he operated on me, he felt that he had somehow 'removed my identity". I presumed that this was because my face would be very different to how it had looked previously. I reassured him that I was a strong woman and that I had a good family and lots of very supportive friends. I completely believed in what I was saying. I was just so relieved that I had had the opportunity to have the operation. He smiled at me and as he left the room, I reflected on what he had shared with me. It filled me with such admiration to think that this intelligent, busy, important man had, whilst I was unconscious, considered the effects of this life changing operation on me as 'a person.' I will remember this conversation for the rest of my life. The compassion evidenced in his words enabled me to fully appreciate the conflicts surgeons face daily and how they truly invest themselves into the care they give to their patients.

My Mother

I struggled however with the reaction from my mother. My father had died many years before and since then, my sister and I had, for various reasons, a difficult relationship with her. Following my diagnosis and treatment she had offered very little in terms of empathy, reassurance or support.

My perception of my mother is that she had always held beauty and wealth in high esteem. She considered herself to be beautiful and had slightly narcissistic personality traits. She was charmed by people who possessed what I considered to be superficial attributes. As children Carol was prettier than me and she was often complimented by members of the family. When Carol and I were young teenager's, my mother took my sister to a local beauty contest and left me at home alone, not perhaps appreciating the effect this had on my level of self-esteem. I remember feeling angry, upset and jealous I suppose. I do not know how I would have reacted if my sister had won. Luckily for me, she did not win but I knew at that moment that my mother did not consider me to be beautiful and it felt like a rejection.

During my recovery Carol, Sharon and I visited my mother and her partner at home. I walked through the lounge and sat at the table with Sharon and my mother was seated on a chair in the lounge area with Carol and my mother's partner. My mother did not acknowledge me or include me in any conversation. She did not ask me how I was feeling or even offer me a drink. As if to compensate she overly exaggerated the conversation she had with Carol enquiring into the activities of her daughter and my mother's grandson in a very disingenuous way. It was very uncomfortable for Carol, Sharon and I and even her partner excused himself to make some refreshments. I should have got up and left. I should have challenged her behaviour because I felt so rejected and upset, but I did as I always have done, I tolerated her conduct. As we left, I heard her quietly ask Sharon how I was! Sharon quite rightly responded: "why don't you ask her?"

There were also instances where my mother would walk into a restaurant and rush round to the other side of the table so that she did not have to sit by me.

I want to believe that my mother may have struggled to cope with my illness and did not want to or could not, accept it. Sadly however, I feel that her ideals and not her emotions affected her behaviour toward me. She was embarrassed about how I looked and preferred to disassociate herself. Despite this, I held no malice towards her. She was my mother and I loved her. She is sadly now deceased, and I miss her.

Despite the hurt I felt at my mother's lack of empathy towards me during this difficult time, she created a forum and welcome distraction for Carol and I to discuss her unusual and often humorous antics. I was under no illusion about the fact that my mother did not consider me to be pretty (although I looked a lot like she had when she was younger!) During one conversation about *"what we would do if we won the lottery"* she interjected, before I had time to respond and asked if I would have a "nose job!" She also considered me to be a little too tall (I am almost six foot) and would attribute every minor ailment such as earache, constipation, in growing toenail (to name a few!) to my height. "Is it because you are so tall?" she would state with the tact of a pre-school aged child. A trip to the hair salon would also give her the opportunity to declare "what have you done to your hair?" My sister and I considered buying her a tea-shirt with "what's wrong with your face?" which was another one of my mother's retorts etched on it but we assumed that she would never wear it.

We offered to take her for lunch most weeks and although, particularly during radiotherapy, I was eating very little, I would enjoy the change of environment. My mother would talk to anyone and her chosen subject would always be about the cruises she had experienced. A simple hello to a stranger whilst waiting at the bar would prompt her to launch into information about her experience on The Queen Mary, Victoria and many other prestigious vessels. My sister and I were in awe of her ability to do this. On one occasion the waitress bought scampi to the table (which was my mother's order). She loudly exclaimed that on the Queen Elizabeth the scampi was much larger, with a lighter coloured coating and that it was offered with an *"array of fine accompaniments"*. As the waitress scurried away, we reminded my mother that we were in fact in a *"Two for Ten"*, rather basic dining establishment and not the QUE2!

Once, whilst out shopping with my mother, I left her browsing in a shoe shop and went next door to a dress shop. I spotted a dress I liked and took it into a changing room to try it on. Several minutes later, I heard my mother calling my name (rather loudly) and questioning where I was. Her voice got shriller as she meandered nearer towards me, and so I had no option but to rather meekly, state my location. With that, she pulled open the dressing room curtain and exposed me, in my underwear, to the rest of the customers in the shop. I grabbed hold of the curtain to help shield myself from the now slightly bemused audience of shoppers and my face went a deep shade of crimson. To add insult to injury my mother entered the changing room took hold of the back of my knickers and tugged them up as she had done when I was about five years old! Oblivious to my acute embarrassment she then handed me an item that she termed a 'pant suit' (which was hideous!) and then stalked off exclaiming that she needed a pair of mauve slacks! For her next cruise! My god! I thought, were we still in the 1970's? I really wished I could have been Mr Ben (an animated character from my childhood) who enters a changing room dressed in a suit and bowler hat. He then opens an imaginary door and ends up in a different country. Unfortunately, I was not Mr Ben! I had to walk out of the shop (past the customers) with my still very red face contrasting hugely against my 'normal' skin coloured prosthetic nose, eye and cheek.

There are many more 'anecdotes' I could include about my mother but the purpose of adding the above is to suggest that; even though I felt that my life was very different, all around me, other people's lives continued as normal. It felt refreshing to be in the company of someone whose life was not compromised or encompassed in the actuality that her daughter, had cancer. It took me some time, but I finally acknowledged, that 'support' can come in many different guises. Whilst out with my mother, it was almost impossible to think about my illness. She invaded my thought processes with her unconventional and often eccentric behaviour and looking retrospectively, this was surprisingly beneficial to my recovery.

10. MY PERCEPTIONS OF ME!

Julie made my first 'proper' prosthesis soon after I was discharged from hospital. It was a similar procedure to a dental impression although of course this was my face and not my teeth. I had to lie back in a therapy chair and gauze was placed into the cavity. A warm liquid was then added, and I had to wait for several minutes until it 'set.' As it hardened it became cold and a little uncomfortable, I had to breathe through my mouth which was uncomfortable as it became dry quite quickly. It was then peeled away to reveal a wax, pink nose, cheek and closed eye. Many other technical procedures had to take place over several weeks before I was able to try the prosthesis on but when I did the prosthesis looked and felt amazing.

As the prosthesis was attached to my face by strong magnets, I was confident that it would remain secure. A small sideways knock, however, would sweep the prosthesis clean off its axis. Luckily, this was a rare occurrence but one day, whilst clearing some space in the conservatory my daughter Emily and I decided to move the sofa. The arm of the sofa hit my nose side on, and the prosthesis 'flew' across the room, bouncing a couple of times before it rested, upward facing by the conservatory doors. We both laughed rather hysterically at this and I think it was then that I realised that I was feeling a little more like my former self.

Within the cavity, the sinuses were still draining and so the discharge would adhere to the middle and sides of the cavity which was composed of mucous membrane. During my recovery, Steve cleaned the cavity for me twice daily, using cotton buds to remove areas of discharge and small plastic instruments to eliminate the more stubborn debris. The cavity was sensitive to touch and the procedure was quite painful and time consuming. Despite this Steve rose to the challenge. He never complained and even when I became a little tearful due to the discomfort, he comforted me or waited for me to compose myself before continuing. I was so relieved that Steve felt comfortable enough to do this for me as the cavity was unsightly and the cleaning procedure difficult. He was not a medical man and yet he seemed completely unphased by the procedure. The discomfort I felt during and after the cleaning process sometimes left me emotionally exhausted, but I knew that it was a small price to pay compared to what the outcome may have been. In time it began to feel more like a routine which we had embedded into our lives and as time passed and I was more able to function with one eye, I managed to clean the cavity myself.

As a child I had never believed that I was particularly pretty, but I could not have imagined the enormity of the impact of losing virtually half of the right side of my face. I almost did not recognise myself, particularly my side profile which of course looked almost flat. I know that many types of cancer can pose body image issues, but the removal of my nose, eye and part of my cheek was something that would be visible for all to see. Sadness and anxiety almost fully consumed me during this time. The sadness was associated with a type of grief and bereavement for the person that I had once been. I 'tortured' myself by looking over old photographs of how I had once looked. Some of the photographs I had once disliked for one reason or another but now I looked at them differently, more intently. I paid attention to the features on my face. My shiny hazel eyes, my slightly freckly nose and my rosy complexion. I looked so pretty and yet I had to accept that I would never look like that again. In addition, I had lost over two and a half stone in weight and I now looked painfully thin and angular making me feel very unfeminine. My neck looked long and thin and my face small, pale and pointed. On a particularly difficult day I told Steve to leave me. I told him that I was no longer the woman he had married and that he could meet someone else who would be physically more attractive. I felt so guilty about how I looked as if it was my own fault. Steve responded well to my anxiety, he had never been an outwardly emotional person but when he spoke his words were meaningful and so very reassuring. He assured me that he loved me as a person and this helped me to gain some perspective. I knew that I would soon have an improved prosthesis and I was still alive!

When I felt more energetic Steve and I would take short trips in the car and visit local beauty spots. I would try to disguise my face as much as possible by wearing sunglasses and a hooded jacket. I would look down to the floor or away from anyone who was passing me in the opposite direction. My confidence was quite low and so I tried anything I could think of to help me to cope.

On one occasion Carol and I went out for a drive. On the way home. we stopped at a convenience store and I entered wearing my sunglasses and the hood which was attached to my coat. As soon as we entered the shop, the shopkeeper who was sitting behind the counter pressed a buzzer. Her husband appeared and asked us, in a quiet voice, to leave the shop. I do not think that Carol had heard him, so we did not leave immediately, we purchased our goods and then exited. As I walked back to Carol's car, I felt upset and discriminated against and wished that I had had the courage to speak out against this seemingly unjust reaction. I felt vulnerable and disliked and this made me very uncomfortable. This experience bought back emotions that I had whilst at school when someone had been unkind to me or I had been criticised or scolded by a teacher. I had lacked resilience then and struggled to manage situations where I perceived that my identity was being compromised. I had been 'protected' whilst I was in hospital as the hospital staff had treated me with kindness and compassion. The hospital had felt like a safe haven, where people would expect to see others looking a little different and readily accept this as part of their health condition. Was this now the new reality for me? Would I have to live a life where I felt that I was being 'judged' and ostracised because of my appearance?

It took me some time to reflect objectively on this situation because I kept reliving it in an almost continuous and cyclical way. I then began to acknowledge the issue from the shopkeeper's perspective. I am almost six foot tall and along with my coat, hood and sunglasses I may have looked odd and alarming. She may have considered that I would be a threat to her personally or that I would have stolen items from her shop. It took some time, but I realised that my 'attempts' to look inconspicuous and preserve the little confidence I had needed to be reconsidered. I instinctively engaged in a series of measures which enabled me to start to accept how I looked and how others may or may not regard me. As summer arrived for example, it became more appropriate to wear sunglasses. They were quite large and covered a considerable section of my face making me feel slightly more self- assured. I had to take them off when I entered a shop or café of course and these short episodes, where I had to reveal my face in public gradually developed into longer periods of time. As both time and occasions progressed and changed, I began to feel a little more confident and comfortable. 'Accept' was not a word I could have used at this time and even whilst writing this there are days when I struggle to 'accept' how I look. On occasion I still mourn for the face I once had.

I was able to talk about my anxieties during my routine appointments with Julie. She offered infinite words of wisdom in that she stated that,

"no member of the public would suspect that you have had lost your nose. People may anticipate that someone could lose their eye but not their nose and part of their cheek".

She informed me that although the prosthetic nose would not completely look like my former nose no-one would ever consider that it was not real. She reminded me also that,

"most people do not look at other people intently. They are too busy going about their normal day".

She asked me if anyone had given me a second glance as I walked into the hospital and I had to admit that they had not. Julie also questioned as to whether (whilst I was in the waiting room) I had seen anyone with a prosthesis and I stated that I had not. She responded by saying that there were two people with prosthetic noses in the waiting room.

Mr Gahir was also very supportive during the follow up consultations. He often commended Steve and I on the cleanliness of the cavity and he commented on how well the prosthesis moulded to my face and its resultant authenticity. His words and his body language encouraged me in a way that no one else really could. He was a 'straight talking man' and I knew that if there was any sort of 'problem', he would tell me about it. Whist his direct approach sometimes added a little to the anxiety I felt as I sat in the waiting room, I always appreciated his honesty and would rather be kept informed. If Mr Gahir was happy with my progress, then I felt that I could relax a little and this added to my overall confidence.

11: CRYING

At least now I could cry. The operation had eradicated the swollen blood vessels from the back of my head and removed the potential for any further bleed. This enabled me to cry and sometimes I would lie on the floor, my body would curl up and my hands would cover the top of my head and hold it tight as if to 'shut out the world'. I would then just cry and cry. The feeling was all encompassing, mentally and physically. Huge sobs would shake my whole body and it was continual, uncontrollable and exhausting. I felt that I could cry for ever. I never felt angry or said, "*why me?*" I never felt jealous of others who were enjoying a healthy life. I just felt so very, very sad. My husband Steve was my 'rock' these during these difficult times, but cancer had created a new, unwelcome chapter in our lives, and he must have felt as shocked and distraught as me. He comforted and supported me with his attention, his touch and his strength. He enabled my recovery and independence by treating me 'normally'. I did not have to pretend that I was coping if I was not. I could be myself and express my emotions positively or negatively as they drifted in and out of my thoughts and he was always there to support me. As time progressed, I felt less overwhelmed and if I did feel like crying, I would do so for a short period of time and then stop and engage myself in something which made me feel happier.

Anxiety was also a problem for me as if I had a headache, increased or different facial pain and soreness I immediately concluded that the cancer had returned. I easily took things out of proportion which was something new to me. I listened intently during each review consultation I had with Mr Gahir and then analysed every word he had said to help reassure myself that I was still well.

I also became quite superstitious, several months before my diagnosis I accidentally broke a large mirror. I had thought fleetingly about the *seven years of bad luck* (an Old Wives tale, supposedly connected with breaking a mirror) but pushed it out of my mind. Despite common sense telling me that this has no relevance to what had happened to me in terms of my health I remain sceptical particularly as seven years have still not passed. I had also purchased a year-long calendar for the study where I wrote in my annual leave and dates of work modules etc. The whole year had been planned out and yet none of it came to fruition. I recall tearing it away from the wall one particularly difficult day and disposing of it rather angrily into a dustbin. I still never write any proposed activities on a calendar or in a diary for fear that something may happen which will prevent me from attending. I suppose I am still a little anxious and this is how such anxiety is manifesting itself.

12: THE MASK

Six weeks after I had recovered from the operation, I faced a huge set back. A CT scan revealed that cerebral spinal fluid was leaking from the skin graft in my head which formed a barrier to my brain. I had to go back to surgery for a minor operation to rectify this problem, but as a result the planned radiotherapy I was to receive was post-phoned for a further six weeks. This created a great deal of distress for me as I was aware that the delay in treatment could increase the chance of the cancer returning and I felt that I may have gone through this major operation for nothing. My mood changed a little during this 'waiting period.' I began to feel a little defeated, I was in 'no man's land,' I missed the support I had always had from Mr Gahir and Julie and there was no other health professional I could talk to during this interim period. This feeling of defeat and increased anxiety temporarily exposed itself in my behaviour and response to others. I became a little irritable and intolerant. A very dear friend visited me one day after I had just received a telephone call from the Cancer Centre at the hospital informing me that I had to attend several appointments, one week apart before I could begin the chemotherapy or radiotherapy. I calculated that this would extend the 'waiting' period to almost sixteen weeks. My friend tried to reassure me, but I was convinced that this delay would result in my demise. My friend had recently lost her mother who she was very close to and she was struggling with grief. She informed me that she had received '*messages*' from her mother as a means I think of comforting me and assuring me that she felt that there 'is life after death.' This information was a little too difficult for me to contemplate and I asked her, quite assertively, to 'stop telling me these things". She apologised profusely but of course she did not need to she was finding it difficult, as I was to comprehend my feelings. On a different occasion another, very dear friend visited me and sensing my 'despair' and 'low mood' asked me if I had '*had a word with myself.*' My friend and I had always enjoyed a rather playful '*say it, as it is*' relationship and I assumed that she was telling me to '*pull myself together.*' Ordinarily I would have accepted her comment and retorted back with something equally as satirical but I was immediately irritated and responded tersely. I apologised of course to both of my friends and realised that I needed to manage the situation I was in, in a more appropriate way. I slowly resigned myself to the fact that there was very little I could do to change things and with this acknowledgement I began to engage in a more positive thought process.

Prior to the radiotherapy I had to have a moulded face mask made. The technician was a lovely man who informed me that the radiotherapy was the '*bib and braces*' (additional support) following the operation. He made it sound so positive, as if I had gone through the worst and this was the part of the journey which would offer me a sense of security. I was asked to lie on the therapeutic couch and a piece of mesh was placed over my face. A substance was then poured over the mesh rather like the procedure for the nose, cheek and eye prosthetic. The cavity was protected from the substance with gauze. The substance felt warm initially but then went cold as it hardened. It felt a little claustrophobic and although I could breathe through my mouth, I was used to the additional air I received through the prosthetic nasal cavity and this was closed off by gauze. As I lay there. I made every attempt to relax by talking to myself inwardly and reassuring myself that it would soon be over. Approximately ten minutes later the mask, which had now hardened, was 'peeled' away from my face. When I looked at the mask, I could see an image of my whole face. I could see the huge voids where my nose, eye and part of my cheek should have been. This highlighted the distortion and asymmetry of my face in a way that I had never seen before and I felt quite alarmed.

Carol had accompanied me to the appointment and had sat some distance away. She had not seen me without my prosthesis, and she told me afterwards that she found it very difficult to accept. She gently explained that she felt that '*I did not look like me anymore*'. I was not upset by her remark. I appreciated her honesty. I needed people to be truthful no matter how difficult it was to hear. It helped me to trust people and their opinions when I was struggling to be sure of my own.

Prior to the chemotherapy and radiotherapy commencing, I met the oncologist. He was a small, serious looking man and he spoke to me in a low melancholic tone. He informed me that I would be having six weeks (thirty sessions). of radiotherapy and two doses of chemotherapy, one at the beginning and one dose after the third week. He seemed pessimistic about the success of the treatment stating that the cancer had been detected at a very late stage and that it was very advanced. The oncologist also appeared unconvinced when the consultant informed him that removing my prosthetic nose for the radiotherapy would be manageable and added instead that the radiotherapy may have to be delivered with the prosthetic nose attached.

The oncologist then enquired as to whether I had any dependent children and I answered that I had not. Initially I thought that he was trying to find out a little more about me and my opinion of him warmed a little. When I got home however, I over analysed his question and to my dismay, I concluded that he may have asked this to ascertain the value of my life in a family where all my adult children were independent.

13: THE AFTER TREATMENT

I had several blood tests to help determine the amount of chemotherapy and radiotherapy my body could cope with without any long -term damage. I also had several more scans to ascertain exactly where the radiotherapy would be directed. There was little room for miscalculation due to the potential damage this may cause to my remaining eye. I also had a consultation with a nurse who informed me that I may lose my hair particularly because the radiotherapy was being directed at my face and forehead. She also explained that I may experience dry skin, facial, mouth and throat sores and that the chemotherapy may make me feel tired and nauseated. At this point I gladly accepted these side effects as I was eager to have the treatment as soon as possible. I reflected on the consultation with the nurse and accepted that whilst I needed to know about the probable side effects of the treatment including the potential for sepsis as the chemotherapy and radiotherapy would reduce my body's ability to 'fight' disease or infections I also considered whether the discussion could have included more positivity. The fact that Carol could accompany me during the chemotherapy, that I would be sitting on a comfortable chair and offered refreshments. She may have included details about the salon at the hospital which offered wigs (if I lost my hair). I am generally a person who is, a 'glass half full' and so I was able to recognise that despite the necessity of the information about the side effects any additional positivity would have been welcome.

Just over fifteen weeks after my major operation the treatment began.

A needle was inserted into my arm and the chemotherapy was commenced. I knew at this point that there was no 'turning back.' The treatment would flow though my veins and enter every part of my body. A young girl sitting opposite to me was struggling with this concept and seemed unsure about having chemotherapy I could empathise with her as whist the purpose of chemotherapy is to be curative, I knew that it could also be very destructive.

Carol and I watched 'Bake off' on my iPad, quietly of course, so as not to disturb others. We laughed at some of the contestants attempts at creating desirable and tasty cuisines although neither of us could have done any better! The three hours were soon over, and I was relieved to think that I only had one more chemotherapy session ahead.

We then had to go to the radiotherapy department. There was a waiting room with approximately fifteen chairs but only three or four people occupying them. They were chatting together, as if they were good friends but I did not feel very sociable and so I sat silently alongside Carol. My name was announced, and the timing was good as my nerves were just beginning to get the better of me. I felt like running towards the exit, but I managed to compose myself. It felt a little like boarding an aeroplane. Just when you realise that you have a slim chance of escape before the stewardess closes the doors and then you are 'trapped.' As you may have already deduced, I am not a fan of flying! I had already had a 'trial run' of the radiotherapy several weeks previously, but this felt very different. This time this 'great silver, grey beast' of a machine would be delivering radium to my face and the effects would be felt throughout my body. Similar, I suppose to the chemotherapy. I knew that both were toxic and destructive yet hopefully curative. I was asked to remove my wig and prosthesis and despite the warmth and friendliness of the radiographers I felt incredibly vulnerable. The little dignity and strength I had was in part, as a result of these adjuncts. I turned away to remove them and stood awkwardly, feeling very exposed. I was invited to lie on the treatment bed, and I was pleasant and responsive, but I offered little eye contact. I think that this was because I was afraid of any visible negative reaction from the radiographers about my facial cavity. I was so acutely sensitive that I would have easily noticed any sign of disdain. I was asked to lie flat, and the 'mask' was placed over my face and 'bolted' somehow into the table. The mask tightened and as the last 'bolt' was secured I could not have moved my head even if I had wanted to.

To add to my feelings of anxiety and as a result of the nature of the surgery, I had a lot of phlegm at the back of my throat, and I was not used to lying flat. I was worried that I would choke because I was unable to cough or sit upright. I was offered a call bell and advised to press it should I need assistance. I then considered that if I were to press the alarm, the radiologists would have to switch off the machine, walk out from behind the radium protective room and free me from the table. How long would this all take? By the time they got to me I would be choking, and perhaps completely hysterical. I knew that I could not let this happen. If I lost control of myself, I would not be able to face having the treatment again and I would be placing my chances of long -term survival into jeopardy. Previous experiences of managing challenging situations such as pain (during childbirth) or fear (launching myself off a water slide called the 'Tsunami' in Greece, (which was clearly not up to British Health and Safety Standards!) was that I became silent. If I had screamed during these times, I would have lost total control of myself and I envisage that I would have to be slapped or sedated before I would regain my composure.

My strategy therefore was to keep my residual eye closed and tax my brain to think of girls' names beginning with the first letter of the alphabet and so on. On another occasion I made up a conversation in French. Unfortunately, at school I had only achieved secondary education level in French language and I am unsure as to how useful 'hello my name is Alison' and 'how many children do you have in your family?' would be. I also made a shopping list (in my head of course!) of food items I needed to order for the week, recounted jokes and recited the alphabet backwards. Despite these less than genius ideas I used to occupy my mind, I could still soon recall every noise the machine made and in which order. I knew when I was halfway through the treatment episode and when it was almost finished. The relief when it was over was tremendous. It did not hurt and only lasted for a few minutes, but it seemed to take forever. Despite the imprint from the mask on my face I was always eager to leave. I thanked the staff, attached my prosthesis and pulled the wig into some sort of position on the top of my head. I would then exit the room to be greeted by my sister who would smile and link my arm as we walked away. As each day and subsequently each week passed, I became more familiar with the people in the waiting room as we were all assigned similar treatment times. I still did not feel the need to speak, but I would smile as I entered and then wave as I exited.

The 'machine' delivering the radiology could easily instil fear into the strongest of people. Despite this I soon began to regard it as my ally, my friend and not my foe. It would hopefully help to save my life. Each session spent lying under this machine was a session nearer to the finish line and hopefully my full recovery. As time progressed, I became more familiar with the radiologists and my feelings of vulnerability reduced considerably. They would always enquire about my well-being and I felt comforted and cared for.

Six weeks, however, soon began to feel like six months and alongside this, I became more unwell. I lost my appetite, felt nauseous and I developed a sore mouth and throat. I was invited to attend weekly appointments with the dietician which helped, and I was given supplements to support my nutrition. My cavity was becoming a little more painful too and so I was prescribed stronger analgesia. Large patches of my hair had fallen out and as a result the wig felt much looser. The facial mask also became a little looser as my face became much thinner. The radiographer discussed the possibility of the need for a new mask but as I only had a week left of treatment it was decided, much to my relief, that this was not necessary. Despite these side effects I had anticipated that I would feel much worse. The soreness in my mouth and throat soon eased, I was given medication for the nausea and this decreased too. The tiredness and loss of appetite persisted for many weeks, but this was something that I was able to manage.

14: MR CHEESE

On one occasion a new individual entered the waiting room. He was about five foot six inches tall and walked with a slight swagger. He greeted everyone and stated his name (which I have now unfortunately forgotten). Carol and I nudged each-other like naughty schoolgirls because we had noticed his tan leather boots which were 'pointy' and folded upwards at the toe making them resemble 'elf shoes.' As he waited, for his appointment, he chatted loudly and indiscriminately about himself. He boasted about how he had made a 'fortune' through his business enabling him to buy fast cars and take luxury holidays. He crowed about his beautiful wife (who had won beauty contests) and the fabulous jewellery he had bought her. The other people in the waiting room would smile, nod, and ooh and ahh! But In contrast, I considered that he had all the charisma of a baboon! Carol and I called him 'Mr Cheese.' The idiom Mr Cheese came from a 1980's 'affliction' thought up by Carol and I. It went alongside Mr 'have one yourself.' In the early 80's my sister and I went to nightclubs together and we could spot these two categories of men a mile off! They were usually; fairly, good looking, short in stature, well dressed (if not a little dated) and full of confidence. Alongside the confidence came the 'tall stories' and boasting behaviours. Mr Cheese would be gushy, full of 'one liner's,' loud and attention seeking. Mr 'have one yourself' would 'flashy' and always carry a wad of cash in his pocket. Whilst ordering drinks at the bar he would vociferously insist that the barperson should 'have one themselves' (hence the name).

The waiting room at the radiotherapy department would slowly empty as people went for their treatments and Carol and I always seemed to be left with 'Mr Cheese.' Whilst there was little opportunity for reciprocal communication (as he monopolised the conversation) I chose to smile and nod at what I thought were appropriate times. I felt no malice towards him only curiosity and silent humour. One day however, much to my combined horror and amusement, I came out from my treatment and Carol was sitting next to him! He beckoned me over to which, for some reason I duly obliged. He then consigned a pained expression on his face. 'I can see that you've had a tough time' he reasoned. '*Mmm,*' I replied. He then stood up, leant forwards and embraced me in a huge bear hug. His strength stopped me from breathing! and his head which was in line with my nose, almost knocked my prosthesis off! He then sat back down and went into detail about his own type of cancer. Whilst listening to his story I began to feel as if I was part of a community. Most of the people who I saw on a weekly basis were either having treatment for cancer or supporting someone with cancer. We had a unique, even if it was slightly detached, bond. I started to feel a fondness for everyone I saw in that room. Each person had their own story and their own worries and fears, even Mr Cheese, who may have needed to chat to people to help him to manage the situation he was in. Carol, (who was still hanging on to his every word) received a frowny, quizzical expression from me and we said our goodbyes and left. Out of sight I reminded her jokily about her current matrimonial commitment and she told me to 'keep my nose out' to which we both laughed hysterically and childishly, pushing and shoving each-other as we left. From then on Mr Cheese's presence at the radiotherapy department became quite comforting. His familiar face and banter helped to reduce my anxiety and make the visits a little more bearable.

During the treatment I had to check my temperature twice daily and on the last week of radiotherapy, my temperature rose to 38 degrees centigrade. I had to ring the cancer centre at the hospital for advice and much to my disappointment

I was advised to attend for a review. I was admitted immediately and given intravenous antibiotics to prevent sepsis as immune system was very low. I had to stay in hospital for a week and in some ways, this was a good thing. I was tiring of the radiotherapy; I found the travel to and from the hospital every weekday tedious and of course I had little energy to build up the motivation to endure the treatment. As I was confined to a hospital bed, I felt that I now had no choice. A porter would arrive at different times each day and wheel me down to the radiotherapy department. The conversations I had with the porter both on the way there and back 'lifted my mood and spirit' and the days seemed to pass by more quickly. On the last day of treatment, I thanked the radiology staff and left them a gift of tea, coffee biscuits and cakes. I was truly grateful for the care and compassion they showed me.

15: HOW DO YOU THANK SOMEONE FOR SAVING YOUR LIFE?

This was something I had thought about time and time again during my recovery. I knew that I would not get the 'all clear' from cancer for several more years but as my short-term prognosis had been so poor, I was grateful to still be alive. I was so thankful to all the consultants involved in my operation, as their combined skills helped to secure my survival. Mr Gahir however, held precedence for me as he was the person who had taken a lead role in my

Surgery, treatment and continued care.

I felt that there was no gift that I could give him which would be big enough or expensive enough to thank him for saving my life. Anything I could give him would seem insignificant against the huge amount of time, effort and expertise he had invested in me.

Following a clear CT scan one day, I asked him if I could hug him, and he said '*yes.*' We both stood up and embraced each other and I simply said, '*thank you, for saving my life.*' Six words that prior to this experience I had never thought that I would ever have to say. I had tears in my eyes, (just as I have writing this) and he looked at me and smiled. Nothing more was said.

I appreciate that whatever happens to me in the future, this lovely, caring and clever man has given all that he has to help me to survive. He also gave me the greatest gift of all and that was to see my daughter Emily get married. I attended wearing a blonde wig and a sensational 'mother of the bride' outfit. Emily asked me to dance the first dance with her and the song was '*Every time you touch me*' by Diana Ross. I had played this to her when she was very young and so it held great meaning for us both.

EPILOGUE

Before I had cancer, I was a life loving, slightly sassy individual who was energetic and spirited. I am still that person, but I am also different.

There is never a day when I feel as 'care- free' as I did before. I suppose this could be because previously I had taken my longevity for granted and I can no longer do this. When I look in a mirror the reflection I see serves as a reminder of a disease that I never thought that I would have and It is hard to forget about when it stares right back at you.

My prosthetic right eye is amazing, but it does not blink or move. My nose has been cast to the shape of my previous nose making it look, incredible. It is not however, *my* nose or eye or part of *my* cheek. It feels hard to the touch, does not change colour (as the rest of my skin does in certain temperatures) and it makes it difficult for me to kiss my husband because it restricts the movement of my mouth.

Despite these issues, I have learned to accept them. I know that I look a little different, but I look OK and I feel happy. If I walk down the street people do not take a second glance at me. Sitting opposite one student nurse or standing in front of huge group of students does not fill me with anxiety anymore. People who did not know me before I had a prosthesis do not know that this is a relatively recent thing for me. They may assume that I have had the prosthesis for many years. People who know me well, tell me that they do not 'see' my prosthesis anymore, it is just a part of 'me'. It *is* part of me! and I am grateful for it. I still take pride in my appearance, apply a little make-up, wear nice clothes and act like a fool sometimes.

I am still alive! And I love my life!